THIS JOURNAL BELONGS TO:

PROGRESS
TRACKER

What to Track	Week 1	Week 2
Weight		
Chest		
Hips		
Arms		
Thighs		

What to Track	Week 3	Week 4	Week 5	Week 6
Weight				
Chest				
Hips				
Arms				
Thighs				

What to Track	Week 7	Week 8	Week 8	Week 10
Weight				
Chest				
Hips				
Arms				
Thighs				

What to Track	Week 11	Week 12	Week 13	Week 14
Weight				
Chest				
Hips				
Arms				
Thighs				

Date: _____ Fasting Day? Y   N

		MACROS	
BREAKFAST		Protein	
		Carbs	
		Fat	
		Calories	
LUNCH		MACROS	
		Protein	
		Carbs	
		Fat	
		Calories	
DINNER		MACROS	
		Protein	
		Carbs	
		Fat	
		Calories	
SNACKS		MACROS	
		Protein	
		Carbs	
		Fat	
		Calories	

Hunger / Cravings

Some

None   Intense

Hydration

Today's Weight

Notes / Observations

....
....
....
....
....
....
....
....
....
....

Today I Feel...

Sleep Quality

Sleep Time

_____

Wake Time

_____

Date: _____ Fasting Day? Y   N

		MACROS	
BREAKFAST		Protein	
		Carbs	
		Fat	
		Calories	
LUNCH		MACROS	
		Protein	
		Carbs	
		Fat	
		Calories	
DINNER		MACROS	
		Protein	
		Carbs	
		Fat	
		Calories	
SNACKS		MACROS	
		Protein	
		Carbs	
		Fat	
		Calories	

Hunger / Cravings

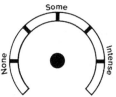

Hydration

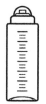

Today's Weight

Notes / Observations

....

....

....

....

....

....

....

....

Today I Feel...

Sleep Quality

Sleep Time

_____

Wake Time

_____

Date: _____   Fasting Day?   Y   N

		MACROS	
BREAKFAST		Protein	
		Carbs	
		Fat	
		Calories	
LUNCH		MACROS	
		Protein	
		Carbs	
		Fat	
		Calories	
DINNER		MACROS	
		Protein	
		Carbs	
		Fat	
		Calories	
SNACKS		MACROS	
		Protein	
		Carbs	
		Fat	
		Calories	

Hunger / Cravings

Some

None   Intense

Hydration

Today's Weight

Notes / Observations

....

....

....

....

....

....

....

....

....

Today I Feel...

Sleep Quality

Sleep Time

_____

Wake Time

_____

Date: _____ Fasting Day?   Y   N

		MACROS	
BREAKFAST		Protein	
		Carbs	
		Fat	
		Calories	
LUNCH		MACROS	
		Protein	
		Carbs	
		Fat	
		Calories	
DINNER		MACROS	
		Protein	
		Carbs	
		Fat	
		Calories	
SNACKS		MACROS	
		Protein	
		Carbs	
		Fat	
		Calories	

Hunger / Cravings

Some

None   Intense

Hydration

Today's Weight

Notes / Observations

....

....

....

....

....

....

....

....

....

....

Today I Feel...

Sleep Quality

Sleep Time

_____

Wake Time

_____

Date: _____ Fasting Day? Y N

		MACROS	
BREAKFAST		Protein	
		Carbs	
		Fat	
		Calories	
LUNCH		MACROS	
		Protein	
		Carbs	
		Fat	
		Calories	
DINNER		MACROS	
		Protein	
		Carbs	
		Fat	
		Calories	
SNACKS		MACROS	
		Protein	
		Carbs	
		Fat	
		Calories	

Hunger / Cravings

Some

None   Intense

Hydration

Today's Weight

Notes / Observations

....

....

....

....

....

....

....

....

....

Today I Feel...

Sleep Quality

Sleep Time

_____

Wake Time

_____

Date: _____   Fasting Day?   Y   N

		MACROS	
BREAKFAST		Protein	
		Carbs	
		Fat	
		Calories	
LUNCH		MACROS	
		Protein	
		Carbs	
		Fat	
		Calories	
DINNER		MACROS	
		Protein	
		Carbs	
		Fat	
		Calories	
SNACKS		MACROS	
		Protein	
		Carbs	
		Fat	
		Calories	

Hunger / Cravings

Some

None   Intense

Hydration

Today's Weight

Notes / Observations

....
....
....
....
....
....
....
....
....
....

Today I Feel...

Sleep Quality

Sleep Time

_____

Wake Time

_____

Date: _____ Fasting Day? Y N

		MACROS	
BREAKFAST		Protein	
		Carbs	
		Fat	
		Calories	
LUNCH		MACROS	
		Protein	
		Carbs	
		Fat	
		Calories	
DINNER		MACROS	
		Protein	
		Carbs	
		Fat	
		Calories	
SNACKS		MACROS	
		Protein	
		Carbs	
		Fat	
		Calories	

Hunger / Cravings

None   Some   Intense

Hydration

Today's Weight

Notes / Observations

....
....
....
....
....
....
....
....
....
....
....
....

Today I Feel...

Sleep Quality

Sleep Time

_____

Wake Time

_____

Date: _____   Fasting Day?   Y   N

		MACROS	
BREAKFAST		Protein	
		Carbs	
		Fat	
		Calories	
LUNCH		MACROS	
		Protein	
		Carbs	
		Fat	
		Calories	
DINNER		MACROS	
		Protein	
		Carbs	
		Fat	
		Calories	
SNACKS		MACROS	
		Protein	
		Carbs	
		Fat	
		Calories	

Hunger / Cravings

Some

None   Intense

Hydration

Today's Weight

Notes / Observations

....
....
....
....
....
....
....
....
....

Today I Feel...

Sleep Quality

Sleep Time

_____

Wake Time

_____

Date: _____ Fasting Day? Y   N

		MACROS	
BREAKFAST		Protein	
		Carbs	
		Fat	
		Calories	
LUNCH		MACROS	
		Protein	
		Carbs	
		Fat	
		Calories	
DINNER		MACROS	
		Protein	
		Carbs	
		Fat	
		Calories	
SNACKS		MACROS	
		Protein	
		Carbs	
		Fat	
		Calories	

Hunger / Cravings

Some

None   Intense

Hydration

Today's Weight

Notes / Observations

....
....
....
....
....
....
....
....
....
....

Today I Feel...

Sleep Quality

Sleep Time

_____

Wake Time

_____

Date: _____   Fasting Day?   Y   N

		MACROS	
BREAKFAST		Protein	
		Carbs	
		Fat	
		Calories	
LUNCH		MACROS	
		Protein	
		Carbs	
		Fat	
		Calories	
DINNER		MACROS	
		Protein	
		Carbs	
		Fat	
		Calories	
SNACKS		MACROS	
		Protein	
		Carbs	
		Fat	
		Calories	

Hunger / Cravings

Some

None   Intense

Hydration

Today's Weight

Notes / Observations

....

....

....

....

....

....

....

....

Today I Feel...

Sleep Quality

Sleep Time

_____

Wake Time

_____

Date: _____   Fasting Day?   Y   N

		MACROS	
BREAKFAST		Protein	
		Carbs	
		Fat	
		Calories	
LUNCH		MACROS	
		Protein	
		Carbs	
		Fat	
		Calories	
DINNER		MACROS	
		Protein	
		Carbs	
		Fat	
		Calories	
SNACKS		MACROS	
		Protein	
		Carbs	
		Fat	
		Calories	

Hunger / Cravings

Some

None   Intense

Hydration

Today's Weight

Notes / Observations

....

....

....

....

....

....

....

....

....

....

....

Today I Feel...

Sleep Quality

Sleep Time

_____

Wake Time

_____

Date: _____ Fasting Day? Y   N

BREAKFAST		Macros	
		Protein	
		Carbs	
		Fat	
		Calories	
LUNCH		Macros	
		Protein	
		Carbs	
		Fat	
		Calories	
DINNER		Macros	
		Protein	
		Carbs	
		Fat	
		Calories	
SNACKS		Macros	
		Protein	
		Carbs	
		Fat	
		Calories	

Hunger / Cravings

Some

None   Intense

Hydration

Today's Weight

Notes / Observations

....
....
....
....
....
....
....
....
....
....
....
....
....
....

Today I Feel...

Sleep Quality

Sleep Time

_____

Wake Time

_____

Date: _____   Fasting Day?   Y   N

		MACROS	
BREAKFAST		Protein	
		Carbs	
		Fat	
		Calories	
LUNCH		MACROS	
		Protein	
		Carbs	
		Fat	
		Calories	
DINNER		MACROS	
		Protein	
		Carbs	
		Fat	
		Calories	
SNACKS		MACROS	
		Protein	
		Carbs	
		Fat	
		Calories	

Hunger / Cravings

Some

None   Intense

Hydration

Today's Weight

Notes / Observations

....
....
....
....
....
....
....
....
....
....

Today I Feel...

Sleep Quality

Sleep Time

_____

Wake Time

_____

Date: _____   Fasting Day?   Y   N

		MACROS	
BREAKFAST		Protein	
		Carbs	
		Fat	
		Calories	
LUNCH		MACROS	
		Protein	
		Carbs	
		Fat	
		Calories	
DINNER		MACROS	
		Protein	
		Carbs	
		Fat	
		Calories	
SNACKS		MACROS	
		Protein	
		Carbs	
		Fat	
		Calories	

Hunger / Cravings

Some
None   Intense

Hydration

Today's Weight

Notes / Observations

....

....

....

....

....

....

....

....

....

....

Today I Feel...

Sleep Quality

Sleep Time

_____

Wake Time

_____

Date: _____   Fasting Day?   Y   N

		MACROS	
BREAKFAST		Protein	
		Carbs	
		Fat	
		Calories	
LUNCH		MACROS	
		Protein	
		Carbs	
		Fat	
		Calories	
DINNER		MACROS	
		Protein	
		Carbs	
		Fat	
		Calories	
SNACKS		MACROS	
		Protein	
		Carbs	
		Fat	
		Calories	

Hunger / Cravings

Some

None   Intense

Hydration

Today's Weight

Notes / Observations

....
....
....
....
....
....
....
....
....
....

Today I Feel...

Sleep Quality

Sleep Time

_____

Wake Time

_____

Date: _____   Fasting Day?   Y   N

		MACROS		Hunger / Cravings
BREAKFAST		Protein		
		Carbs		
		Fat		
		Calories		
LUNCH		MACROS		
		Protein		Hydration
		Carbs		
		Fat		
		Calories		
DINNER		MACROS		
		Protein		
		Carbs		
		Fat		
		Calories		Today's Weight
SNACKS		MACROS		
		Protein		
		Carbs		
		Fat		
		Calories		

Notes / Observations

....

....

....

....

....

....

....

....

Today I Feel...

Sleep Quality

Sleep Time

_____

Wake Time

_____

Date: _____   Fasting Day?   Y   N

	MACROS	
BREAKFAST	Protein	
	Carbs	
	Fat	
	Calories	
	MACROS	
LUNCH	Protein	
	Carbs	
	Fat	
	Calories	
	MACROS	
DINNER	Protein	
	Carbs	
	Fat	
	Calories	
	MACROS	
SNACKS	Protein	
	Carbs	
	Fat	
	Calories	

Hunger / Cravings

None   Some   Intense

Hydration

Today's Weight

Notes / Observations

....
....
....
....
....
....
....
....
....
....

Today I Feel...

Sleep Quality

Sleep Time

_____

Wake Time

_____

Date: _____   Fasting Day?   Y   N

		MACROS	
BREAKFAST		Protein	
		Carbs	
		Fat	
		Calories	
LUNCH		MACROS	
		Protein	
		Carbs	
		Fat	
		Calories	
DINNER		MACROS	
		Protein	
		Carbs	
		Fat	
		Calories	
SNACKS		MACROS	
		Protein	
		Carbs	
		Fat	
		Calories	

Hunger / Cravings

Some

None   Intense

Hydration

Today's Weight

Notes / Observations

....

....

....

....

....

....

....

....

Today I Feel...

Sleep Quality

Sleep Time

_____

Wake Time

_____

Date: _____ Fasting Day?   Y   N

	MACROS		Hunger / Cravings
BREAKFAST	Protein		
	Carbs		
	Fat		
	Calories		
	MACROS		
LUNCH	Protein		Hydration
	Carbs		
	Fat		
	Calories		
	MACROS		
DINNER	Protein		
	Carbs		
	Fat		
	Calories		Today's Weight
	MACROS		
SNACKS	Protein		
	Carbs		
	Fat		
	Calories		

Notes / Observations

....
....
....
....
....
....
....
....
....
....
....
....

Today I Feel...

Sleep Quality

Sleep Time

_____

Wake Time

_____

Date: _____   Fasting Day?   Y   N

		MACROS	
BREAKFAST		Protein	
		Carbs	
		Fat	
		Calories	
LUNCH		MACROS	
		Protein	
		Carbs	
		Fat	
		Calories	
DINNER		MACROS	
		Protein	
		Carbs	
		Fat	
		Calories	
SNACKS		MACROS	
		Protein	
		Carbs	
		Fat	
		Calories	

Hunger / Cravings

Some

None   Intense

Hydration

Today's Weight

Notes / Observations

....
....
....
....
....
....
....
....
....

Today I Feel...

Sleep Quality

Sleep Time

_____

Wake Time

_____

Date: _____ Fasting Day?   Y   N

		MACROS		Hunger / Cravings
BREAKFAST		Protein		
		Carbs		
		Fat		
		Calories		
LUNCH		MACROS		
		Protein		Hydration
		Carbs		
		Fat		
		Calories		
DINNER		MACROS		
		Protein		
		Carbs		
		Fat		
		Calories		Today's Weight
SNACKS		MACROS		
		Protein		
		Carbs		
		Fat		
		Calories		

Notes / Observations

....
....
....
....
....
....
....
....
....
....
....

Today I Feel...

Sleep Quality

Sleep Time

_____

Wake Time

_____

Date: _____ Fasting Day? Y N

		MACROS	
BREAKFAST		Protein	
		Carbs	
		Fat	
		Calories	
LUNCH		MACROS	
		Protein	
		Carbs	
		Fat	
		Calories	
DINNER		MACROS	
		Protein	
		Carbs	
		Fat	
		Calories	
SNACKS		MACROS	
		Protein	
		Carbs	
		Fat	
		Calories	

Hunger / Cravings

Some

None   Intense

Hydration

Today's Weight

Notes / Observations

....

....

....

....

....

....

....

....

....

Today I Feel...

Sleep Quality

Sleep Time

_____

Wake Time

_____

Date: _____   Fasting Day?   Y   N

	MACROS	
BREAKFAST	Protein	
	Carbs	
	Fat	
	Calories	

Hunger / Cravings

	MACROS	
LUNCH	Protein	
	Carbs	
	Fat	
	Calories	

Hydration

	MACROS	
DINNER	Protein	
	Carbs	
	Fat	
	Calories	

Today's Weight

	MACROS	
SNACKS	Protein	
	Carbs	
	Fat	
	Calories	

Notes / Observations

....
....
....
....
....
....
....
....
....
....
....

Today I Feel...

Sleep Quality

Sleep Time

_____

Wake Time

_____

Date: _____ Fasting Day?   Y   N

		MACROS	
BREAKFAST		Protein	
		Carbs	
		Fat	
		Calories	
LUNCH		MACROS	
		Protein	
		Carbs	
		Fat	
		Calories	
DINNER		MACROS	
		Protein	
		Carbs	
		Fat	
		Calories	
SNACKS		MACROS	
		Protein	
		Carbs	
		Fat	
		Calories	

Hunger / Cravings

Some

None   Intense

Hydration

Today's Weight

Notes / Observations

....

....

....

....

....

....

....

....

....

....

....

....

Today I Feel...

Sleep Quality

Sleep Time

_____

Wake Time

_____

Date: _____   Fasting Day?   Y   N

	MACROS	
BREAKFAST	Protein	
	Carbs	
	Fat	
	Calories	
	MACROS	
LUNCH	Protein	
	Carbs	
	Fat	
	Calories	
	MACROS	
DINNER	Protein	
	Carbs	
	Fat	
	Calories	
	MACROS	
SNACKS	Protein	
	Carbs	
	Fat	
	Calories	

Hunger / Cravings

Some
None   Intense

Hydration

Today's Weight

Notes / Observations

....
....
....
....
....
....
....
....
....

Today I Feel...

Sleep Quality

Sleep Time

_____

Wake Time

_____

Date: _____   Fasting Day?   Y   N

		MACROS	
BREAKFAST		Protein	
		Carbs	
		Fat	
		Calories	
LUNCH		MACROS	
		Protein	
		Carbs	
		Fat	
		Calories	
DINNER		MACROS	
		Protein	
		Carbs	
		Fat	
		Calories	
SNACKS		MACROS	
		Protein	
		Carbs	
		Fat	
		Calories	

Hunger / Cravings

Some

None   Intense

Hydration

Today's Weight

Notes / Observations

....
....
....
....
....
....
....
....
....
....
....

Today I Feel...

Sleep Quality

Sleep Time

_____

Wake Time

_____

Date: _____ Fasting Day?   Y   N

		MACROS	
BREAKFAST		Protein	
		Carbs	
		Fat	
		Calories	
LUNCH		MACROS	
		Protein	
		Carbs	
		Fat	
		Calories	
DINNER		MACROS	
		Protein	
		Carbs	
		Fat	
		Calories	
SNACKS		MACROS	
		Protein	
		Carbs	
		Fat	
		Calories	

Hunger / Cravings

Some

None   Intense

Hydration

Today's Weight

Notes / Observations

Today I Feel...

Sleep Quality

Sleep Time

_____

Wake Time

_____

Date: _____ Fasting Day?   Y   N

		MACROS	
BREAKFAST		Protein	
		Carbs	
		Fat	
		Calories	
LUNCH		MACROS	
		Protein	
		Carbs	
		Fat	
		Calories	
DINNER		MACROS	
		Protein	
		Carbs	
		Fat	
		Calories	
SNACKS		MACROS	
		Protein	
		Carbs	
		Fat	
		Calories	

Hunger / Cravings

None   Some   Intense

Hydration

Today's Weight

Notes / Observations

....

....

....

....

....

....

....

....

....

Today I Feel...

Sleep Quality

Sleep Time

_____

Wake Time

_____

Date: _____   Fasting Day?   Y   N

		MACROS	
BREAKFAST		Protein	
		Carbs	
		Fat	
		Calories	
LUNCH		MACROS	
		Protein	
		Carbs	
		Fat	
		Calories	
DINNER		MACROS	
		Protein	
		Carbs	
		Fat	
		Calories	
SNACKS		MACROS	
		Protein	
		Carbs	
		Fat	
		Calories	

Hunger / Cravings

Some

None   Intense

Hydration

Today's Weight

Notes / Observations

....
....
....
....
....
....
....
....
....
....
....
....

Today I Feel...

Sleep Quality

Sleep Time
_____

Wake Time
_____

Date: _____   Fasting Day?   Y   N

		MACROS	
BREAKFAST		Protein	
		Carbs	
		Fat	
		Calories	
LUNCH		MACROS	
		Protein	
		Carbs	
		Fat	
		Calories	
DINNER		MACROS	
		Protein	
		Carbs	
		Fat	
		Calories	
SNACKS		MACROS	
		Protein	
		Carbs	
		Fat	
		Calories	

Hunger / Cravings

Some

None   Intense

Hydration

Today's Weight

Notes / Observations

....
....
....
....
....
....
....
....
....
....
....

Today I Feel...

Sleep Quality

Sleep Time

_____

Wake Time

_____

Date: _____   Fasting Day?   Y   N

		MACROS	
BREAKFAST		Protein	
		Carbs	
		Fat	
		Calories	
LUNCH		MACROS	
		Protein	
		Carbs	
		Fat	
		Calories	
DINNER		MACROS	
		Protein	
		Carbs	
		Fat	
		Calories	
SNACKS		MACROS	
		Protein	
		Carbs	
		Fat	
		Calories	

Hunger / Cravings

Some
None   Intense

Hydration

Today's Weight

Notes / Observations

....
....
....
....
....
....
....
....
....
....
....

Today I Feel...

Sleep Quality

Sleep Time

_____

Wake Time

_____

Date: _____   Fasting Day?   Y   N

		MACROS	
BREAKFAST		Protein	
		Carbs	
		Fat	
		Calories	
LUNCH		MACROS	
		Protein	
		Carbs	
		Fat	
		Calories	
DINNER		MACROS	
		Protein	
		Carbs	
		Fat	
		Calories	
SNACKS		MACROS	
		Protein	
		Carbs	
		Fat	
		Calories	

Hunger / Cravings

Some

None   Intense

Hydration

Today's Weight

Notes / Observations

....

....

....

....

....

....

....

....

....

....

....

Today I Feel...

Sleep Quality

Sleep Time

_____

Wake Time

_____

Date: _____ Fasting Day?   Y   N

	MACROS		Hunger / Cravings
BREAKFAST	Protein		
	Carbs		
	Fat		
	Calories		
LUNCH	MACROS		Hydration
	Protein		
	Carbs		
	Fat		
	Calories		
DINNER	MACROS		
	Protein		
	Carbs		
	Fat		
	Calories		Today's Weight
SNACKS	MACROS		
	Protein		
	Carbs		
	Fat		
	Calories		

Notes / Observations

....

....

....

....

....

....

....

....

....

....

....

Today I Feel...

Sleep Quality

Sleep Time

_____

Wake Time

_____

Date: _____   Fasting Day?   Y   N

		MACROS	
BREAKFAST		Protein	
		Carbs	
		Fat	
		Calories	
LUNCH		MACROS	
		Protein	
		Carbs	
		Fat	
		Calories	
DINNER		MACROS	
		Protein	
		Carbs	
		Fat	
		Calories	
SNACKS		MACROS	
		Protein	
		Carbs	
		Fat	
		Calories	

Hunger / Cravings

Some

None   Intense

Hydration

Today's Weight

Notes / Observations

....

....

....

....

....

....

....

....

Today I Feel...

Sleep Quality

Sleep Time

_____

Wake Time

_____

Date: _____   Fasting Day?   Y   N

BREAKFAST		MACROS	
		Protein	
		Carbs	
		Fat	
		Calories	
LUNCH		MACROS	
		Protein	
		Carbs	
		Fat	
		Calories	
DINNER		MACROS	
		Protein	
		Carbs	
		Fat	
		Calories	
SNACKS		MACROS	
		Protein	
		Carbs	
		Fat	
		Calories	

Hunger / Cravings

Some

None   Intense

Hydration

Today's Weight

Notes / Observations

Today I Feel...

Sleep Quality

Sleep Time

_____

Wake Time

_____

Date: _____   Fasting Day?   Y   N

		MACROS	
BREAKFAST		Protein	
		Carbs	
		Fat	
		Calories	
LUNCH		MACROS	
		Protein	
		Carbs	
		Fat	
		Calories	
DINNER		MACROS	
		Protein	
		Carbs	
		Fat	
		Calories	
SNACKS		MACROS	
		Protein	
		Carbs	
		Fat	
		Calories	

Hunger / Cravings

Some

None   Intense

Hydration

Today's Weight

Notes / Observations

....

....

....

....

....

....

....

....

....

Today I Feel...

Sleep Quality

Sleep Time

_____

Wake Time

_____

Date: _____ Fasting Day?   Y   N

		MACROS	
BREAKFAST		Protein	
		Carbs	
		Fat	
		Calories	
LUNCH		MACROS	
		Protein	
		Carbs	
		Fat	
		Calories	
DINNER		MACROS	
		Protein	
		Carbs	
		Fat	
		Calories	
SNACKS		MACROS	
		Protein	
		Carbs	
		Fat	
		Calories	

Hunger / Cravings

Some

None

Intense

Hydration

Today's Weight

Notes / Observations

....

....

....

....

....

....

....

....

....

....

Today I Feel...

Sleep Quality

Sleep Time

_____

Wake Time

_____

Date: _____   Fasting Day?   Y   N

		MACROS	
BREAKFAST		Protein	
		Carbs	
		Fat	
		Calories	
LUNCH		MACROS	
		Protein	
		Carbs	
		Fat	
		Calories	
DINNER		MACROS	
		Protein	
		Carbs	
		Fat	
		Calories	
SNACKS		MACROS	
		Protein	
		Carbs	
		Fat	
		Calories	

Hunger / Cravings

Some

None   Intense

Hydration

Today's Weight

Notes / Observations

....

....

....

....

....

....

....

....

Today I Feel...

Sleep Quality

Sleep Time

_____

Wake Time

_____

Date: _____   Fasting Day?   Y   N

	MACROS	
BREAKFAST	Protein	
	Carbs	
	Fat	
	Calories	
	MACROS	
LUNCH	Protein	
	Carbs	
	Fat	
	Calories	
	MACROS	
DINNER	Protein	
	Carbs	
	Fat	
	Calories	
	MACROS	
SNACKS	Protein	
	Carbs	
	Fat	
	Calories	

Hunger / Cravings

Some

None

Intense

Hydration

Today's Weight

Notes / Observations

Today I Feel...

Sleep Quality

Sleep Time

_____

Wake Time

_____

Date: _____   Fasting Day?   Y   N

		MACROS	
BREAKFAST		Protein	
		Carbs	
		Fat	
		Calories	
LUNCH		MACROS	
		Protein	
		Carbs	
		Fat	
		Calories	
DINNER		MACROS	
		Protein	
		Carbs	
		Fat	
		Calories	
SNACKS		MACROS	
		Protein	
		Carbs	
		Fat	
		Calories	

Hunger / Cravings

Some

None   Intense

Hydration

Today's Weight

Notes / Observations

....
....
....
....
....
....
....
....

Today I Feel...

Sleep Quality

Sleep Time

_____

Wake Time

_____

Date: _____   Fasting Day?   Y   N

	MACROS	
BREAKFAST	Protein	
	Carbs	
	Fat	
	Calories	
	MACROS	
LUNCH	Protein	
	Carbs	
	Fat	
	Calories	
	MACROS	
DINNER	Protein	
	Carbs	
	Fat	
	Calories	
	MACROS	
SNACKS	Protein	
	Carbs	
	Fat	
	Calories	

Hunger / Cravings

Hydration

Today's Weight

Notes / Observations

....
....
....
....
....
....
....
....
....
....
....
....

Today I Feel...

Sleep Quality

Sleep Time

_____

Wake Time

_____

Date: _____ Fasting Day?   Y   N

BREAKFAST		MACROS	
		Protein	
		Carbs	
		Fat	
		Calories	

LUNCH		MACROS	
		Protein	
		Carbs	
		Fat	
		Calories	

DINNER		MACROS	
		Protein	
		Carbs	
		Fat	
		Calories	

SNACKS		MACROS	
		Protein	
		Carbs	
		Fat	
		Calories	

Hunger / Cravings

Some

None   Intense

Hydration

Today's Weight

Notes / Observations

....
....
....
....
....
....
....
....
....
....

Today I Feel...

Sleep Quality

Sleep Time

_____

Wake Time

_____

Date: _____   Fasting Day?   Y   N

		MACROS	
BREAKFAST		Protein	
		Carbs	
		Fat	
		Calories	
LUNCH		MACROS	
		Protein	
		Carbs	
		Fat	
		Calories	
DINNER		MACROS	
		Protein	
		Carbs	
		Fat	
		Calories	
SNACKS		MACROS	
		Protein	
		Carbs	
		Fat	
		Calories	

Hunger / Cravings

Hydration

Today's Weight

Notes / Observations

....
....
....
....
....
....
....
....
....
....
....

Today I Feel...

Sleep Quality

Sleep Time

_____

Wake Time

_____

Date: _____   Fasting Day?   Y   N

		MACROS	
BREAKFAST		Protein	
		Carbs	
		Fat	
		Calories	
LUNCH		MACROS	
		Protein	
		Carbs	
		Fat	
		Calories	
DINNER		MACROS	
		Protein	
		Carbs	
		Fat	
		Calories	
SNACKS		MACROS	
		Protein	
		Carbs	
		Fat	
		Calories	

Hunger / Cravings

Some

None   Intense

Hydration

Today's Weight

Notes / Observations

....
....
....
....
....
....
....
....
....

Today I Feel...

Sleep Quality

Sleep Time

_____

Wake Time

_____

Date: _____   Fasting Day?   Y   N

		MACROS	
BREAKFAST		Protein	
		Carbs	
		Fat	
		Calories	
LUNCH		MACROS	
		Protein	
		Carbs	
		Fat	
		Calories	
DINNER		MACROS	
		Protein	
		Carbs	
		Fat	
		Calories	
SNACKS		MACROS	
		Protein	
		Carbs	
		Fat	
		Calories	

Hunger / Cravings

Some

None   Intense

Hydration

Today's Weight

Notes / Observations

....

....

....

....

....

....

....

....

....

....

Today I Feel...

Sleep Quality

Sleep Time

_____

Wake Time

_____

Date: _____ Fasting Day?   Y   N

		MACROS	
BREAKFAST		Protein	
		Carbs	
		Fat	
		Calories	
LUNCH		MACROS	
		Protein	
		Carbs	
		Fat	
		Calories	
DINNER		MACROS	
		Protein	
		Carbs	
		Fat	
		Calories	
SNACKS		MACROS	
		Protein	
		Carbs	
		Fat	
		Calories	

Hunger / Cravings

Some

None

Intense

Hydration

Today's Weight

Notes / Observations

....
....
....
....
....
....
....
....
....

Today I Feel...

Sleep Quality

Sleep Time

_____

Wake Time

_____

Date: _____   Fasting Day?   Y   N

BREAKFAST		MACROS	
		Protein	
		Carbs	
		Fat	
		Calories	

Hunger / Cravings

LUNCH		MACROS	
		Protein	
		Carbs	
		Fat	
		Calories	

Hydration

DINNER		MACROS	
		Protein	
		Carbs	
		Fat	
		Calories	

Today's Weight

SNACKS		MACROS	
		Protein	
		Carbs	
		Fat	
		Calories	

Notes / Observations

....
....
....
....
....
....
....
....
....
....

Today I Feel...

Sleep Quality

Sleep Time

_____

Wake Time

_____

Date: _____ Fasting Day? Y   N

BREAKFAST		MACROS	
		Protein	
		Carbs	
		Fat	
		Calories	
LUNCH		MACROS	
		Protein	
		Carbs	
		Fat	
		Calories	
DINNER		MACROS	
		Protein	
		Carbs	
		Fat	
		Calories	
SNACKS		MACROS	
		Protein	
		Carbs	
		Fat	
		Calories	

Hunger / Cravings

Some

None   Intense

Hydration

Today's Weight

Notes / Observations

....

....

....

....

....

....

....

....

....

....

....

Today I Feel...

Sleep Quality

Sleep Time

_____

Wake Time

_____

Date: _____   Fasting Day?   Y   N

	MACROS	
BREAKFAST	Protein	
	Carbs	
	Fat	
	Calories	
	MACROS	
LUNCH	Protein	
	Carbs	
	Fat	
	Calories	
	MACROS	
DINNER	Protein	
	Carbs	
	Fat	
	Calories	
	MACROS	
SNACKS	Protein	
	Carbs	
	Fat	
	Calories	

Hunger / Cravings

Hydration

Today's Weight

Notes / Observations

....
....
....
....
....
....
....
....
....
....
....
....
....

Today I Feel...

Sleep Quality

Sleep Time

_____

Wake Time

_____

Date: _____ Fasting Day? Y   N

BREAKFAST		MACROS	
		Protein	
		Carbs	
		Fat	
		Calories	
LUNCH		MACROS	
		Protein	
		Carbs	
		Fat	
		Calories	
DINNER		MACROS	
		Protein	
		Carbs	
		Fat	
		Calories	
SNACKS		MACROS	
		Protein	
		Carbs	
		Fat	
		Calories	

Hunger / Cravings

None   Some   Intense

Hydration

Today's Weight

Notes / Observations

....
....
....
....
....
....
....
....
....
....

Today I Feel...

Sleep Quality

Sleep Time

_____

Wake Time

_____

Date: _____ Fasting Day? Y   N

		MACROS	
BREAKFAST		Protein	
		Carbs	
		Fat	
		Calories	
LUNCH		MACROS	
		Protein	
		Carbs	
		Fat	
		Calories	
DINNER		MACROS	
		Protein	
		Carbs	
		Fat	
		Calories	
SNACKS		MACROS	
		Protein	
		Carbs	
		Fat	
		Calories	

Hunger / Cravings

Some

None   Intense

Hydration

Today's Weight

Notes / Observations

....
....
....
....
....
....
....
....
....
....
....

Today I Feel...

Sleep Quality

Sleep Time

_____

Wake Time

_____

Date: _____   Fasting Day?   Y   N

BREAKFAST		MACROS	
		Protein	
		Carbs	
		Fat	
		Calories	
LUNCH		MACROS	
		Protein	
		Carbs	
		Fat	
		Calories	
DINNER		MACROS	
		Protein	
		Carbs	
		Fat	
		Calories	
SNACKS		MACROS	
		Protein	
		Carbs	
		Fat	
		Calories	

Hunger / Cravings

None   Some   Intense

Hydration

Today's Weight

Notes / Observations

....

....

....

....

....

....

....

....

....

Today I Feel...

Sleep Quality

Sleep Time

_____

Wake Time

_____

Date: _____   Fasting Day?   Y   N

	MACROS	
BREAKFAST	Protein	
	Carbs	
	Fat	
	Calories	
	MACROS	
LUNCH	Protein	
	Carbs	
	Fat	
	Calories	
	MACROS	
DINNER	Protein	
	Carbs	
	Fat	
	Calories	
	MACROS	
SNACKS	Protein	
	Carbs	
	Fat	
	Calories	

Hunger / Cravings

None   Some   Intense

Hydration

Today's Weight

Notes / Observations

....
....
....
....
....
....
....
....
....
....
....
....

Today I Feel...

Sleep Quality

Sleep Time

_____

Wake Time

_____

Date: _____   Fasting Day?   Y   N

		MACROS	
BREAKFAST		Protein	
		Carbs	
		Fat	
		Calories	
LUNCH		MACROS	
		Protein	
		Carbs	
		Fat	
		Calories	
DINNER		MACROS	
		Protein	
		Carbs	
		Fat	
		Calories	
SNACKS		MACROS	
		Protein	
		Carbs	
		Fat	
		Calories	

Hunger / Cravings

Some

None   Intense

Hydration

Today's Weight

Notes / Observations

....
....
....
....
....
....
....
....
....

Today I Feel...

Sleep Quality

Sleep Time

_____

Wake Time

_____

Date: _____   Fasting Day?   Y   N

BREAKFAST		MACROS	
		Protein	
		Carbs	
		Fat	
		Calories	
LUNCH		MACROS	
		Protein	
		Carbs	
		Fat	
		Calories	
DINNER		MACROS	
		Protein	
		Carbs	
		Fat	
		Calories	
SNACKS		MACROS	
		Protein	
		Carbs	
		Fat	
		Calories	

Hunger / Cravings

Some

None   Intense

Hydration

Today's Weight

Notes / Observations

....
....
....
....
....
....
....
....
....
....

Today I Feel...

Sleep Quality

Sleep Time
_____

Wake Time
_____

Date: _____ Fasting Day?   Y   N

		MACROS	
BREAKFAST		Protein	
		Carbs	
		Fat	
		Calories	
LUNCH		MACROS	
		Protein	
		Carbs	
		Fat	
		Calories	
DINNER		MACROS	
		Protein	
		Carbs	
		Fat	
		Calories	
SNACKS		MACROS	
		Protein	
		Carbs	
		Fat	
		Calories	

Hunger / Cravings

Some

None   Intense

Hydration

Today's Weight

Notes / Observations

....

....

....

....

....

....

....

....

....

Today I Feel...

Sleep Quality

Sleep Time

_____

Wake Time

_____

z^Z_z

Date: _____   Fasting Day?   Y   N

	MACROS		Hunger / Cravings
BREAKFAST	Protein		
	Carbs		
	Fat		
	Calories		
	MACROS		
LUNCH	Protein		Hydration
	Carbs		
	Fat		
	Calories		
	MACROS		
DINNER	Protein		
	Carbs		
	Fat		
	Calories		Today's Weight
	MACROS		
SNACKS	Protein		
	Carbs		
	Fat		
	Calories		

Notes / Observations

....
....
....
....
....
....
....
....
....
....
....
....
....

Today I Feel...

Sleep Quality

Sleep Time

_____

Wake Time

_____

Date: _____ Fasting Day?   Y   N

		MACROS		Hunger / Cravings
BREAKFAST		Protein		
		Carbs		
		Fat		
		Calories		
LUNCH		MACROS		Hydration
		Protein		
		Carbs		
		Fat		
		Calories		
DINNER		MACROS		
		Protein		
		Carbs		
		Fat		
		Calories		Today's Weight
SNACKS		MACROS		
		Protein		
		Carbs		
		Fat		
		Calories		

Notes / Observations

....

....

....

....

....

....

....

....

Today I Feel...

Sleep Quality

Sleep Time

_____

Wake Time

_____

Date: _____ Fasting Day?   Y   N

		MACROS		Hunger / Cravings
BREAKFAST		Protein		
		Carbs		
		Fat		
		Calories		
LUNCH		MACROS		Hydration
		Protein		
		Carbs		
		Fat		
		Calories		
DINNER		MACROS		
		Protein		
		Carbs		
		Fat		
		Calories		Today's Weight
SNACKS		MACROS		
		Protein		
		Carbs		
		Fat		
		Calories		

Notes / Observations

....

....

....

....

....

....

....

....

....

Today I Feel...

Sleep Quality

Sleep Time

_____

Wake Time

_____

Date: _____   Fasting Day?   Y   N

		MACROS	
BREAKFAST		Protein	
		Carbs	
		Fat	
		Calories	
LUNCH		MACROS	
		Protein	
		Carbs	
		Fat	
		Calories	
DINNER		MACROS	
		Protein	
		Carbs	
		Fat	
		Calories	
SNACKS		MACROS	
		Protein	
		Carbs	
		Fat	
		Calories	

Hunger / Cravings

Some

None · Intense

Hydration

Today's Weight

Notes / Observations

....
....
....
....
....
....
....
....
....
....

Today I Feel...

Sleep Quality

Sleep Time

_____

Wake Time

_____

Date: _____   Fasting Day?   Y   N

	MACROS		Hunger / Cravings
BREAKFAST	Protein		
	Carbs		
	Fat		
	Calories		
	MACROS		
LUNCH	Protein		Hydration
	Carbs		
	Fat		
	Calories		
	MACROS		
DINNER	Protein		
	Carbs		
	Fat		
	Calories		Today's Weight
	MACROS		
SNACKS	Protein		
	Carbs		
	Fat		
	Calories		

Notes / Observations

....
....
....
....
....
....
....
....
....
....
....

Today I Feel...

Sleep Quality

Sleep Time

_____

Wake Time

_____

Date: _____   Fasting Day?   Y   N

		MACROS	
BREAKFAST		Protein	
		Carbs	
		Fat	
		Calories	
LUNCH		MACROS	
		Protein	
		Carbs	
		Fat	
		Calories	
DINNER		MACROS	
		Protein	
		Carbs	
		Fat	
		Calories	
SNACKS		MACROS	
		Protein	
		Carbs	
		Fat	
		Calories	

Hunger / Cravings

Some

None   Intense

Hydration

Today's Weight

Notes / Observations

....
....
....
....
....
....
....
....

Today I Feel...

Sleep Quality

Sleep Time

_____

Wake Time

_____

Date: _____ Fasting Day? Y   N

	MACROS	
BREAKFAST	Protein	
	Carbs	
	Fat	
	Calories	
	MACROS	
LUNCH	Protein	
	Carbs	
	Fat	
	Calories	
	MACROS	
DINNER	Protein	
	Carbs	
	Fat	
	Calories	
	MACROS	
SNACKS	Protein	
	Carbs	
	Fat	
	Calories	

Hunger / Cravings

Some

None   Intense

Hydration

Today's Weight

Notes / Observations

Today I Feel...

Sleep Quality

Sleep Time

_____

Wake Time

_____

Date: _____   Fasting Day?   Y   N

BREAKFAST		MACROS	
		Protein	
		Carbs	
		Fat	
		Calories	
LUNCH		MACROS	
		Protein	
		Carbs	
		Fat	
		Calories	
DINNER		MACROS	
		Protein	
		Carbs	
		Fat	
		Calories	
SNACKS		MACROS	
		Protein	
		Carbs	
		Fat	
		Calories	

Hunger / Cravings

Some

None   Intense

Hydration

Today's Weight

Notes / Observations

....
....
....
....
....
....
....
....
....

Today I Feel...

Sleep Quality

Sleep Time

_____

Wake Time

_____

Date: _____ Fasting Day?   Y   N

		MACROS		Hunger / Cravings
BREAKFAST		Protein		Some
		Carbs		
		Fat		None / Intense
		Calories		
LUNCH		MACROS		
		Protein		Hydration
		Carbs		
		Fat		
		Calories		
DINNER		MACROS		
		Protein		
		Carbs		
		Fat		
		Calories		Today's Weight
SNACKS		MACROS		
		Protein		
		Carbs		
		Fat		
		Calories		

Notes / Observations

....
....
....
....
....
....
....
....
....

Today I Feel...

Sleep Quality

Sleep Time

_____

Wake Time

_____

Date: _____   Fasting Day?   Y   N

BREAKFAST		MACROS	
		Protein	
		Carbs	
		Fat	
		Calories	
LUNCH		MACROS	
		Protein	
		Carbs	
		Fat	
		Calories	
DINNER		MACROS	
		Protein	
		Carbs	
		Fat	
		Calories	
SNACKS		MACROS	
		Protein	
		Carbs	
		Fat	
		Calories	

Hunger / Cravings

Some
None   Intense

Hydration

Today's Weight

Notes / Observations

....
....
....
....
....
....
....
....
....
....
....
....

Today I Feel...

Sleep Quality

Sleep Time

_____

Wake Time

_____

Date: _____   Fasting Day?   Y   N

		MACROS	
BREAKFAST		Protein	
		Carbs	
		Fat	
		Calories	
LUNCH		MACROS	
		Protein	
		Carbs	
		Fat	
		Calories	
DINNER		MACROS	
		Protein	
		Carbs	
		Fat	
		Calories	
SNACKS		MACROS	
		Protein	
		Carbs	
		Fat	
		Calories	

Hunger / Cravings

Some
None   Intense

Hydration

Today's Weight

Notes / Observations

....
....
....
....
....
....
....
....
....
....
....
....
....
....
....
....

Today I Feel...

Sleep Quality

Sleep Time

_____

Wake Time

_____

Date: _____   Fasting Day?   Y   N

BREAKFAST		Macros	
		Protein	
		Carbs	
		Fat	
		Calories	
LUNCH		Macros	
		Protein	
		Carbs	
		Fat	
		Calories	
DINNER		Macros	
		Protein	
		Carbs	
		Fat	
		Calories	
SNACKS		Macros	
		Protein	
		Carbs	
		Fat	
		Calories	

Hunger / Cravings

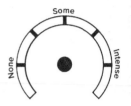

Hydration

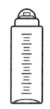

Today's Weight

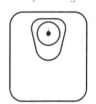

Notes / Observations

....

....

....

....

....

....

....

....

Today I Feel...

Sleep Quality

Sleep Time

_____

Wake Time

_____

Date: _____   Fasting Day?   Y   N

		MACROS	
BREAKFAST		Protein	
		Carbs	
		Fat	
		Calories	
LUNCH		MACROS	
		Protein	
		Carbs	
		Fat	
		Calories	
DINNER		MACROS	
		Protein	
		Carbs	
		Fat	
		Calories	
SNACKS		MACROS	
		Protein	
		Carbs	
		Fat	
		Calories	

Hunger / Cravings

None   Some   Intense

Hydration

Today's Weight

Notes / Observations

....
....
....
....
....
....
....
....
....
....

Today I Feel...

Sleep Quality

Sleep Time

_____

Wake Time

_____

Date: _____   Fasting Day?   Y   N

		MACROS	
BREAKFAST		Protein	
		Carbs	
		Fat	
		Calories	
LUNCH		MACROS	
		Protein	
		Carbs	
		Fat	
		Calories	
DINNER		MACROS	
		Protein	
		Carbs	
		Fat	
		Calories	
SNACKS		MACROS	
		Protein	
		Carbs	
		Fat	
		Calories	

Hunger / Cravings

Some

None   Intense

Hydration

Today's Weight

Notes / Observations

....
....
....
....
....
....
....
....

Today I Feel...

Sleep Quality

Sleep Time

_____

Wake Time

_____

Date: _____   Fasting Day?   Y   N

BREAKFAST		MACROS	
		Protein	
		Carbs	
		Fat	
		Calories	
LUNCH		MACROS	
		Protein	
		Carbs	
		Fat	
		Calories	
DINNER		MACROS	
		Protein	
		Carbs	
		Fat	
		Calories	
SNACKS		MACROS	
		Protein	
		Carbs	
		Fat	
		Calories	

Hunger / Cravings

Hydration

Today's Weight

Notes / Observations

....
....
....
....
....
....
....
....
....
....

Today I Feel...

Sleep Quality

Sleep Time

_____

Wake Time

_____

Date: _____   Fasting Day?   Y   N

		MACROS	
BREAKFAST		Protein	
		Carbs	
		Fat	
		Calories	
LUNCH		MACROS	
		Protein	
		Carbs	
		Fat	
		Calories	
DINNER		MACROS	
		Protein	
		Carbs	
		Fat	
		Calories	
SNACKS		MACROS	
		Protein	
		Carbs	
		Fat	
		Calories	

Hunger / Cravings

Some

None   Intense

Hydration

Today's Weight

Notes / Observations

....
....
....
....
....
....
....
....
....

Today I Feel...

Sleep Quality

Sleep Time

_____

Wake Time

_____

Date: _____   Fasting Day? Y   N

		MACROS	
BREAKFAST		Protein	
		Carbs	
		Fat	
		Calories	
LUNCH		MACROS	
		Protein	
		Carbs	
		Fat	
		Calories	
DINNER		MACROS	
		Protein	
		Carbs	
		Fat	
		Calories	
SNACKS		MACROS	
		Protein	
		Carbs	
		Fat	
		Calories	

Hunger / Cravings

Some
None   Intense

Hydration

Today's Weight

Notes / Observations

....
....
....
....
....
....
....
....
....
....

Today I Feel...

Sleep Quality

Sleep Time

_____

Wake Time

_____

Date: _____   Fasting Day?   Y   N

	MACROS	
BREAKFAST	Protein	
	Carbs	
	Fat	
	Calories	
	MACROS	
LUNCH	Protein	
	Carbs	
	Fat	
	Calories	
	MACROS	
DINNER	Protein	
	Carbs	
	Fat	
	Calories	
	MACROS	
SNACKS	Protein	
	Carbs	
	Fat	
	Calories	

Hunger / Cravings

Some

None   Intense

Hydration

Today's Weight

Notes / Observations

....

....

....

....

....

....

....

....

Today I Feel...

Sleep Quality

Sleep Time

_____

Wake Time

_____

Date: _____   Fasting Day?   Y   N

		MACROS	
BREAKFAST		Protein	
		Carbs	
		Fat	
		Calories	
LUNCH		MACROS	
		Protein	
		Carbs	
		Fat	
		Calories	
DINNER		MACROS	
		Protein	
		Carbs	
		Fat	
		Calories	
SNACKS		MACROS	
		Protein	
		Carbs	
		Fat	
		Calories	

Hunger / Cravings

Some

None   Intense

Hydration

Today's Weight

Notes / Observations

....
....
....
....
....
....
....
....
....

Today I Feel...

Sleep Quality

Sleep Time

_____

Wake Time

_____

Date: _____   Fasting Day?   Y   N

		MACROS	
BREAKFAST		Protein	
		Carbs	
		Fat	
		Calories	
LUNCH		MACROS	
		Protein	
		Carbs	
		Fat	
		Calories	
DINNER		MACROS	
		Protein	
		Carbs	
		Fat	
		Calories	
SNACKS		MACROS	
		Protein	
		Carbs	
		Fat	
		Calories	

Hunger / Cravings

Some

None   Intense

Hydration

Today's Weight

Notes / Observations

....
....
....
....
....
....
....
....
....

Today I Feel...

Sleep Quality

Sleep Time

_____

Wake Time

_____

Date: _____   Fasting Day?   Y   N

	MACROS		Hunger / Cravings
BREAKFAST	Protein		
	Carbs		
	Fat		
	Calories		

	MACROS		
LUNCH	Protein		Hydration
	Carbs		
	Fat		
	Calories		

	MACROS		
DINNER	Protein		
	Carbs		
	Fat		
	Calories		Today's Weight

	MACROS		
SNACKS	Protein		
	Carbs		
	Fat		
	Calories		

Notes / Observations

....

....

....

....

....

....

....

....

....

....

Today I Feel...

Sleep Quality

Sleep Time

_____

Wake Time

_____

Date: _____ Fasting Day?   Y   N

		MACROS	
BREAKFAST		Protein	
		Carbs	
		Fat	
		Calories	
LUNCH		MACROS	
		Protein	
		Carbs	
		Fat	
		Calories	
DINNER		MACROS	
		Protein	
		Carbs	
		Fat	
		Calories	
SNACKS		MACROS	
		Protein	
		Carbs	
		Fat	
		Calories	

Hunger / Cravings

Some
None   Intense

Hydration

Today's Weight

Notes / Observations

....
....
....
....
....
....
....
....
....
....
....
....
....

Today I Feel...

Sleep Quality

Sleep Time

_____

Wake Time

_____

Date: _____   Fasting Day?   Y   N

		MACROS		Hunger / Cravings
BREAKFAST		Protein		
		Carbs		
		Fat		
		Calories		
LUNCH		MACROS		
		Protein		Hydration
		Carbs		
		Fat		
		Calories		
DINNER		MACROS		
		Protein		
		Carbs		
		Fat		
		Calories		Today's Weight
SNACKS		MACROS		
		Protein		
		Carbs		
		Fat		
		Calories		

Notes / Observations

....

....

....

....

....

....

....

....

....

....

Today I Feel...

Sleep Quality

Sleep Time

_____

Wake Time

_____

Date: _____   Fasting Day?   Y   N

		MACROS	
BREAKFAST		Protein	
		Carbs	
		Fat	
		Calories	
LUNCH		MACROS	
		Protein	
		Carbs	
		Fat	
		Calories	
DINNER		MACROS	
		Protein	
		Carbs	
		Fat	
		Calories	
SNACKS		MACROS	
		Protein	
		Carbs	
		Fat	
		Calories	

Hunger / Cravings

Hydration

Today's Weight

Notes / Observations

....

....

....

....

....

....

....

....

....

....

....

Today I Feel...

Sleep Quality

Sleep Time

_____

Wake Time

_____

Date: _____   Fasting Day?   Y   N

		MACROS	
BREAKFAST		Protein	
		Carbs	
		Fat	
		Calories	
LUNCH		MACROS	
		Protein	
		Carbs	
		Fat	
		Calories	
DINNER		MACROS	
		Protein	
		Carbs	
		Fat	
		Calories	
SNACKS		MACROS	
		Protein	
		Carbs	
		Fat	
		Calories	

Hunger / Cravings

None   Some   Intense

Hydration

Today's Weight

Notes / Observations

....
....
....
....
....
....
....
....
....

Today I Feel...

Sleep Quality

Sleep Time

_____

Wake Time

_____

Date: _____   Fasting Day?   Y   N

		MACROS	
BREAKFAST		Protein	
		Carbs	
		Fat	
		Calories	
LUNCH		MACROS	
		Protein	
		Carbs	
		Fat	
		Calories	
DINNER		MACROS	
		Protein	
		Carbs	
		Fat	
		Calories	
SNACKS		MACROS	
		Protein	
		Carbs	
		Fat	
		Calories	

Hunger / Cravings

Some

None   Intense

Hydration

Today's Weight

Notes / Observations

....
....
....
....
....
....
....
....

Today I Feel...

Sleep Quality

Sleep Time

_____

Wake Time

_____

Date: _____   Fasting Day?   Y   N

	MACROS	
BREAKFAST	Protein	
	Carbs	
	Fat	
	Calories	
	MACROS	
LUNCH	Protein	
	Carbs	
	Fat	
	Calories	
	MACROS	
DINNER	Protein	
	Carbs	
	Fat	
	Calories	
	MACROS	
SNACKS	Protein	
	Carbs	
	Fat	
	Calories	

Hunger / Cravings

Some
None   Intense

Hydration

Today's Weight

Notes / Observations

....
....
....
....
....
....
....
....
....
....

Today I Feel...

Sleep Quality

Sleep Time

_____

Wake Time

_____

Date: _____   Fasting Day?   Y   N

BREAKFAST		MACROS	
		Protein	
		Carbs	
		Fat	
		Calories	
LUNCH		MACROS	
		Protein	
		Carbs	
		Fat	
		Calories	
DINNER		MACROS	
		Protein	
		Carbs	
		Fat	
		Calories	
SNACKS		MACROS	
		Protein	
		Carbs	
		Fat	
		Calories	

Hunger / Cravings

Some
None   Intense

Hydration

Today's Weight

Notes / Observations

....

....

....

....

....

....

....

....

....

....

Today I Feel...

Sleep Quality

Sleep Time

_____

Wake Time

_____

Date: _____   Fasting Day?   Y   N

BREAKFAST		MACROS	
		Protein	
		Carbs	
		Fat	
		Calories	
LUNCH		MACROS	
		Protein	
		Carbs	
		Fat	
		Calories	
DINNER		MACROS	
		Protein	
		Carbs	
		Fat	
		Calories	
SNACKS		MACROS	
		Protein	
		Carbs	
		Fat	
		Calories	

Hunger / Cravings

Some

None   Intense

Hydration

Today's Weight

Notes / Observations

....

....

....

....

....

....

....

....

....

Today I Feel...

Sleep Quality

Sleep Time

_____

Wake Time

_____

Date: _____   Fasting Day?   Y   N

		MACROS	
BREAKFAST		Protein	
		Carbs	
		Fat	
		Calories	
LUNCH		MACROS	
		Protein	
		Carbs	
		Fat	
		Calories	
DINNER		MACROS	
		Protein	
		Carbs	
		Fat	
		Calories	
SNACKS		MACROS	
		Protein	
		Carbs	
		Fat	
		Calories	

Hunger / Cravings

Some
None   Intense

Hydration

Today's Weight

Notes / Observations

....
....
....
....
....
....
....
....
....
....

Today I Feel...

Sleep Quality

Sleep Time

_____

Wake Time

_____

Date: _____   Fasting Day?   Y   N

	MACROS		Hunger / Cravings
BREAKFAST	Protein		
	Carbs		
	Fat		
	Calories		
	MACROS		
LUNCH	Protein		Hydration
	Carbs		
	Fat		
	Calories		
	MACROS		
DINNER	Protein		
	Carbs		
	Fat		
	Calories		Today's Weight
	MACROS		
SNACKS	Protein		
	Carbs		
	Fat		
	Calories		

Notes / Observations

....

....

....

....

....

....

....

....

....

....

....

....

Today I Feel...

Sleep Quality

Sleep Time

_____

Wake Time

_____

Date: _____   Fasting Day?   Y   N

		MACROS	
BREAKFAST		Protein	
		Carbs	
		Fat	
		Calories	
LUNCH		MACROS	
		Protein	
		Carbs	
		Fat	
		Calories	
DINNER		MACROS	
		Protein	
		Carbs	
		Fat	
		Calories	
SNACKS		MACROS	
		Protein	
		Carbs	
		Fat	
		Calories	

Hunger / Cravings

Some

None   Intense

Hydration

Today's Weight

Notes / Observations

....

....

....

....

....

....

....

....

....

Today I Feel...

Sleep Quality

Sleep Time

_____

Wake Time

_____

Date: _____   Fasting Day?   Y   N

BREAKFAST		MACROS	
		Protein	
		Carbs	
		Fat	
		Calories	

Hunger / Cravings

Some

None   Intense

LUNCH		MACROS	
		Protein	
		Carbs	
		Fat	
		Calories	

Hydration

DINNER		MACROS	
		Protein	
		Carbs	
		Fat	
		Calories	

Today's Weight

SNACKS		MACROS	
		Protein	
		Carbs	
		Fat	
		Calories	

Notes / Observations

....
....
....
....
....
....
....
....
....
....

Today I Feel...

Sleep Quality

Sleep Time

_____

Wake Time

_____

Date: _____   Fasting Day?   Y   N

		MACROS	
BREAKFAST		Protein	
		Carbs	
		Fat	
		Calories	
LUNCH		MACROS	
		Protein	
		Carbs	
		Fat	
		Calories	
DINNER		MACROS	
		Protein	
		Carbs	
		Fat	
		Calories	
SNACKS		MACROS	
		Protein	
		Carbs	
		Fat	
		Calories	

Hunger / Cravings

Some

None   Intense

Hydration

Today's Weight

Notes / Observations

....
....
....
....
....
....
....
....

Today I Feel...

Sleep Quality

Sleep Time

_____

Wake Time

_____

Date: _____   Fasting Day?   Y   N

	MACROS	
BREAKFAST	Protein	
	Carbs	
	Fat	
	Calories	
	MACROS	
LUNCH	Protein	
	Carbs	
	Fat	
	Calories	
	MACROS	
DINNER	Protein	
	Carbs	
	Fat	
	Calories	
	MACROS	
SNACKS	Protein	
	Carbs	
	Fat	
	Calories	

Hunger / Cravings

Hydration

Today's Weight

Notes / Observations

....
....
....
....
....
....
....
....
....
....

Today I Feel...

Sleep Quality

Sleep Time

_____

Wake Time

_____

Date: _____   Fasting Day?   Y   N

		MACROS	
BREAKFAST		Protein	
		Carbs	
		Fat	
		Calories	
LUNCH		MACROS	
		Protein	
		Carbs	
		Fat	
		Calories	
DINNER		MACROS	
		Protein	
		Carbs	
		Fat	
		Calories	
SNACKS		MACROS	
		Protein	
		Carbs	
		Fat	
		Calories	

Hunger / Cravings

Hydration

Today's Weight

Notes / Observations

....

....

....

....

....

....

....

....

....

Today I Feel...

Sleep Quality

Sleep Time

_____

Wake Time

_____

Date: _____   Fasting Day?   Y   N

		MACROS	
BREAKFAST		Protein	
		Carbs	
		Fat	
		Calories	
LUNCH		MACROS	
		Protein	
		Carbs	
		Fat	
		Calories	
DINNER		MACROS	
		Protein	
		Carbs	
		Fat	
		Calories	
SNACKS		MACROS	
		Protein	
		Carbs	
		Fat	
		Calories	

Hunger / Cravings

Some

None   Intense

Hydration

Today's Weight

Notes / Observations

....
....
....
....
....
....
....
....
....
....
....
....

Today I Feel...

Sleep Quality

Sleep Time

_____

Wake Time

_____

Date: _____   Fasting Day?   Y   N

		MACROS	
BREAKFAST		Protein	
		Carbs	
		Fat	
		Calories	
LUNCH		MACROS	
		Protein	
		Carbs	
		Fat	
		Calories	
DINNER		MACROS	
		Protein	
		Carbs	
		Fat	
		Calories	
SNACKS		MACROS	
		Protein	
		Carbs	
		Fat	
		Calories	

Hunger / Cravings

None   Some   Intense

Hydration

Today's Weight

Notes / Observations

....

....

....

....

....

....

....

....

Today I Feel...

Sleep Quality

Sleep Time

_____

Wake Time

_____

Date: _____   Fasting Day?   Y   N

	MACROS	
BREAKFAST	Protein	
	Carbs	
	Fat	
	Calories	
	MACROS	
LUNCH	Protein	
	Carbs	
	Fat	
	Calories	
	MACROS	
DINNER	Protein	
	Carbs	
	Fat	
	Calories	
	MACROS	
SNACKS	Protein	
	Carbs	
	Fat	
	Calories	

Hunger / Cravings

Some

None   Intense

Hydration

Today's Weight

Notes / Observations

....

....

....

....

....

....

....

....

....

....

Today I Feel...

Sleep Quality

Sleep Time

_____

Wake Time

_____

Date: _____ Fasting Day?   Y   N

		MACROS	
BREAKFAST		Protein	
		Carbs	
		Fat	
		Calories	
LUNCH		MACROS	
		Protein	
		Carbs	
		Fat	
		Calories	
DINNER		MACROS	
		Protein	
		Carbs	
		Fat	
		Calories	
SNACKS		MACROS	
		Protein	
		Carbs	
		Fat	
		Calories	

Hunger / Cravings

Some

None   Intense

Hydration

Today's Weight

Notes / Observations

....
....
....
....
....
....
....
....
....
....
....
....

Today I Feel...

Sleep Quality

Sleep Time

_____

Wake Time

_____

Date: _____ Fasting Day? Y N

		MACROS	
BREAKFAST		Protein	
		Carbs	
		Fat	
		Calories	
LUNCH		MACROS	
		Protein	
		Carbs	
		Fat	
		Calories	
DINNER		MACROS	
		Protein	
		Carbs	
		Fat	
		Calories	
SNACKS		MACROS	
		Protein	
		Carbs	
		Fat	
		Calories	

Hunger / Cravings

Some
None   Intense

Hydration

Today's Weight

Notes / Observations

....
....
....
....
....
....
....
....
....
....

Today I Feel...

Sleep Quality

Sleep Time

_____

Wake Time

_____

Date: _____   Fasting Day?   Y   N

		MACROS	
BREAKFAST		Protein	
		Carbs	
		Fat	
		Calories	
LUNCH		MACROS	
		Protein	
		Carbs	
		Fat	
		Calories	
DINNER		MACROS	
		Protein	
		Carbs	
		Fat	
		Calories	
SNACKS		MACROS	
		Protein	
		Carbs	
		Fat	
		Calories	

Hunger / Cravings

Some

None   Intense

Hydration

Today's Weight

Notes / Observations

....

....

....

....

....

....

....

....

Today I Feel...

Sleep Quality

Sleep Time

_____

Wake Time

_____

Date: _____ Fasting Day?   Y   N

	MACROS	
BREAKFAST	Protein	
	Carbs	
	Fat	
	Calories	
	MACROS	
LUNCH	Protein	
	Carbs	
	Fat	
	Calories	
	MACROS	
DINNER	Protein	
	Carbs	
	Fat	
	Calories	
	MACROS	
SNACKS	Protein	
	Carbs	
	Fat	
	Calories	

Hunger / Cravings

Hydration

Today's Weight

Notes / Observations

....

....

....

....

....

....

....

....

....

....

....

Today I Feel...

Sleep Quality

Sleep Time

_____

Wake Time

_____

Made in the USA
Columbia, SC
17 March 2021